LOW SODIUM FOOD LIST AND COOKBOOK FOR ADULTS

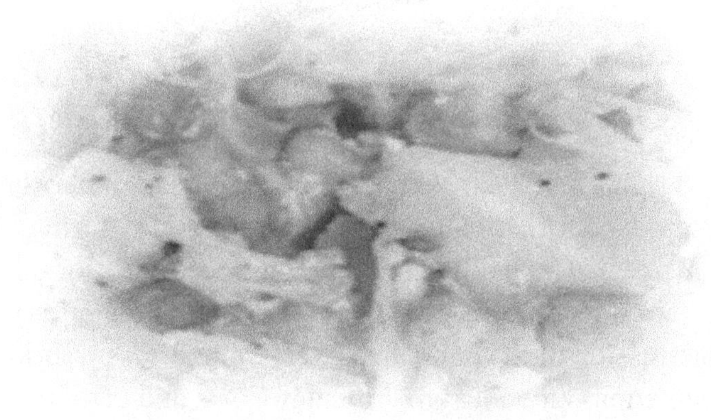

Comprehensive Guide to Low Sodium Foods and Recipes For Healthy Living.

David T. Salcedo

TABLE OF CONTENTS

INTRODUCTION

Alex Turner an adult with an uncommon commitment to health, lived in the dynamic metropolis, where the pace of life matched the rhythm of its streets. His road to a low salt lifestyle began not with a famous tale, but with the awareness that his health demanded more attention than the city's never-ending hustle permitted.

As a software engineer caught up in a flurry of deadlines and late-night coding sessions, Alex was confronted with the implications of an unregulated diet. High salt levels were doing havoc on his health, buried in the convenience of takeout meals and office snacks. Alex felt he had to make a change when his doctor offered a severe warning during a routine exam.

His transition was not an overnight makeover, but rather a progressive evolution. Alex began by visiting the city's farmers' markets, where he discovered the brilliant colors and flavors of fresh, low sodium vegetables. Fruits and vegetables were his allies, replacing the manufactured foods that had previously dominated his workstation.

Alex had to become a culinary explorer in order to embrace a low sodium diet. He began on a voyage through his own kitchen, armed with herbs and spices instead of a salt shaker, experimenting with recipes that converted bland into assertive. Quinoa salads, grilled fish with lemon zest, and colorful stir-fries became his signature meals, indicating a shift away from his sodium-laden background.

Dining out became an art form for Alex, who developed her skills by asking questions, requesting changes, and selecting places that appreciated the necessity of health-conscious meals. Rather than feeling constrained, he found joy in exploring new flavors that enhanced rather than hid the essence of each dish.

Alex's dedication was no longer jeopardized by social events. He confidently traversed the sea of party platters and restaurant spreads, armed with information and a sense of purpose. His buddies, initially perplexed by the lack of a salt shaker, quickly accepted the refreshing alteration, learning that flavor does not have to be sacrificed for the sake of health.

Alex found himself not only healthier but happy as the seasons changed and Metropolis bustled with its customary vitality. His was not a fairy tale with magical potions, but rather a demonstration of the transformational power of deliberate choices. Alex Turner lived a vibrant, low sodium symphony in the middle of the city—an homage to well-being and the pursuit of a better, heartier tomorrow.

WHAT IS SODIUM

Sodium has the symbol Na and the atomic number 11. It is a highly reactive alkali metal that belongs to the periodic table's alkali metal group. Sodium is a soft, silver-white metal with a low melting point. It is so reactive that it is never discovered in nature in its elemental form, but rather in diverse compounds.

Sodium chloride, a common table salt, is one of the most well-known sodium compounds. Sodium is essential in many biological functions, including fluid balance management, neuronal transmission, and muscle contraction. While sodium is necessary for health, excessive sodium consumption, generally in the form of salt, has been linked to health hazards such as high blood pressure, heart disease, and stroke.

In terms of dietary advice, health professionals frequently recommend lowering sodium intake to maintain general health. This guidance has resulted in a greater awareness of the salt level in processed foods, as well as the encouragement of low-sodium diets for those looking to lower their risk of certain health disorders.

Importance of Low Sodium on Health

A Low sodium diet is critical for overall health and the prevention of different chronic illnesses. When ingested in excess, sodium, a mineral necessary for human activities, can have negative effects. Here's a detailed examination of the significance of a low salt diet:

1. Blood Pressure Regulation

The most well-known advantage of a Low sodium diet is its ability to lower blood pressure. Excess sodium consumption has been related to high blood pressure (hypertension), a key risk factor for heart disease and stroke.

Reducing salt helps the body maintain a better fluid balance, which helps regulate blood pressure levels.

2. Cardiovascular Health

A Low sodium diet contributes to cardiovascular health by minimizing the strain on the heart and blood vessels. It reduces the chance of developing diseases like heart disease, heart attacks, and strokes.

People who already have cardiovascular disease may benefit from a Low sodium diet as part of a complete management plan.

3. Kidney Function

The kidneys play an important function in managing salt balance in the body. A Low sodium diet helps minimize kidney disease by reducing the workload on the kidneys.

A Low sodium diet may be recommended for patients with kidney disorders or compromised kidney function to manage their condition and slow the course of kidney damage

4. Fluid Balance and Edema Prevention

Sodium affects the fluid balance of the body. A low sodium diet reduces swelling in numerous regions of the body by preventing fluid retention and edema.

This is especially critical for people who have diseases like heart failure, when fluid retention can exacerbate symptoms.

5. Osteoporosis Prevention

A high sodium intake is linked to increased calcium excretion in the urine, which may contribute to lower bone density. A Low sodium diet may aid in the prevention of osteoporosis and the preservation of bone health.

6. Reduced Risk of Stroke

Hypertension, which is commonly associated with high sodium intake, is a substantial risk factor for strokes. Individuals can reduce their risk of both ischemic and hemorrhagic strokes by controlling their blood pressure with a reduced salt diet.

7. Improved Arterial Health

Excess sodium can contribute to artery stiffness, increasing the burden on the heart. A Low sodium diet improves arterial health by lowering the risk of atherosclerosis and other vascular problems.

8. Positive Impact on Cognitive Function

Some research reveals a possible link between high salt consumption and cognitive deterioration. Individuals who follow a reduced salt diet may support greater cognitive function and lower their risk of neurological disorders.

9. Weight Management

Processed and high-sodium foods are frequently connected with higher calorie content. A low sodium diet that emphasizes fresh, natural foods can help with weight management and overall health.

10. Long-Term Health and Disease Prevention

Adopting a reduced salt diet is a preventive step for preventing chronic diseases that can develop over time. Dietary patterns, including salt intake, may influence conditions such as cardiovascular disease, kidney issues, and some types of cancer.

11. Pregnancy Health

Maintaining a good sodium balance throughout pregnancy is critical for preventing diseases such as gestational hypertension and preeclampsia. A Low sodium dietmay be recommended to promote a healthy pregnancy.

12. Promoting Overall Well-Being

Aside from specific health concerns, a reduced salt diet improves overall well-being. It promotes the eating of nutrient-dense, whole foods that deliver necessary vitamins and minerals without the additional health hazards associated with excessive salt consumption.

RECOMMENDED DAILY SODIUM INTAKE

The basic guidelines for salt intake are as follows, according to the Dietary Guidelines for Americans 2020-2025, issued by the United States Departments of Health and Human Services (HHS) and Agriculture (USDA):

• Adults should aim for less than 2,300 milligrams (mg) of sodium per day; for certain population groups, such as those 51 and older, African Americans, and those with hypertension, diabetes, or chronic kidney disease, the recommended limit is reduced to 1,500 mg per day.

These recommendations are intended to promote cardiovascular health and lower the risk of problems such as hypertension (high blood pressure) and cardiovascular disease. It's crucial to know that processed and packaged foods typically include a considerable amount of salt, so being careful of food choices and reading labels can help with sodium management.

Individuals with certain health concerns, as well as those under the care of a healthcare expert, may obtain individualized advice suited to their specific health needs. Always seek counsel from your healthcare professional or a certified dietitian for advice tailored to your personal health state and needs. Furthermore, requirements may differ by country, therefore it is critical to consult the precise instructions offered by health authorities in your region.

HEALTH RISK ASSOCIATED WITH HIGH SODIUM INTAKE

High salt intake is linked to several health problems, especially when it surpasses recommended levels. The chief health hazards connected with excessive salt consumption are as follows:

1. High Blood Pressure (Hypertension)

- Hypertension is one of the most well-known health hazards associated with increased sodium intake. Because sodium draws water, an excess of sodium in the bloodstream can cause an increase in blood volume, placing pressure on blood vessels.
- Persistently high blood pressure can harm arteries, contribute to atherosclerosis (artery hardening), and increase the risk of heart disease, stroke, and other cardiovascular problems.

2. Cardiovascular Diseases

- Hypertension caused by high sodium intake is a major risk factor for cardiovascular diseases such as coronary artery disease, heart attacks, and heart failure.

- The increased workload on the heart and damage to blood vessels contribute to the overall deterioration of cardiovascular health.

3. Stroke

- High blood pressure, which is frequently associated with excessive sodium consumption, is a significant cause of strokes. Strokes happen when blood arteries in the brain become damaged or obstructed, disrupting blood flow and oxygen supply to the brain.

4. Kidney Damage

- Kidney damage is important because the kidneys regulate salt balance. High sodium levels can strain the kidneys and contribute to renal damage over time. • People who already have kidney problems may be more vulnerable to the negative effects of high salt intake.

5. Fluid Retention and Edema

- Because salt draws water, an excess of sodium consumption can cause fluid retention, resulting in swelling or edema, particularly in the extremities.
- Fluid retention can exacerbate conditions such as heart failure, further jeopardizing health.

6. Osteoporosis

- Some studies suggest a link between high sodium intake and increased calcium excretion through urine, potentially leading to decreased bone density.
- This calcium loss may contribute to the development of osteoporosis, a condition characterized by weakened and brittle bones, over time.

7. Cognitive Decline

- New research suggests a possible link between high salt intake and cognitive decline. Excess salt may have a deleterious impact on neurological health and cognitive function, but further research is needed to determine the precise pathways.

8. Stomach Cancer

- A high salt diet, frequently in the form of salt-preserved foods, has been linked to an increased risk of stomach cancer.

- The World Health Organization (WHO) recognized a link between excessive salt consumption and the development of stomach cancer.

9. Exacerbation of Other Conditions

- High sodium intake may aggravate certain health disorders, such as asthma and Meniere's disease, due to its effect on fluid balance and inflammation.

10. Overall Impact on Public Health

- The cumulative health impacts of high sodium intake contribute to a considerable public health burden, resulting in greater healthcare expenses and a higher prevalence of chronic diseases.

11. Impaired Arterial Function

- Excess sodium can lead to arterial stiffness, impairing blood vessel expansion and contraction. This impairment might cause blood pressure to rise even higher and put strain on the cardiovascular system.

12. Increased Risk During Pregnancy

- High sodium consumption during pregnancy may contribute to gestational hypertension and preeclampsia, offering dangers to both the mother and the unborn child.

LOW SODIUM FOOD LIST

Fruits and vegetables

Fruits

1. Apples

2. Bananas

3. Berries (Strawberries, Blueberries, Raspberries)

4. Peaches

5. Plums

6. Watermelon

7. Cantaloupe

8. Oranges

9. Grapes

10. Kiwi

11. Pineapple

12. Mango

13. Pears

14. Cherries

15. Papaya

16. Cranberries

17. Apricots

18. Figs

19. Grapefruit

20. Avocado

Vegetables

21. Spinach

22. Kale

23. Broccoli

24. Cauliflower

25. Carrots

26. Bell Peppers

27. Cucumbers

28. Zucchini

29. Sweet Potatoes

30. Asparagus

Lean Proteins

1. **Skinless Chicken Breast:** A versatile and lean source of protein.

2. **Turkey Breast:** Another lean poultry option with lower sodium content.

3. **Fish (Salmon, Cod, Haddock):** Rich in omega-3 fatty acids and protein.

4. **Tuna (Fresh or Canned in Water):** A convenient and protein-packed option.

5. **Shrimp:** Low in fat and calories, shrimp is a good source of protein.

6. **Lean Ground Turkey:** A lower-fat alternative to ground beef.

7. **Lean Ground Chicken:** Versatile and lower in saturated fat.

8. **Egg Whites:** Pure protein without the cholesterol found in yolks.

9. **Greek Yogurt (Non-fat or Low-fat):** Higher protein content compared to regular yogurt.

10. **Cottage Cheese (Low-fat):** A dairy option with a good protein-to-calorie ratio.

11. **Tofu:** A plant-based protein source suitable for various dishes.

12. **Tempeh:** A fermented soy product with a nutty flavor.

13. **Edamame:** Young soybeans that can be enjoyed as a snack or added to dishes.

14. **Lentils:** A legume rich in protein, fiber, and various nutrients.

15. **Chickpeas:** Versatile and protein-rich legumes.

16. **Black Beans:** A good source of plant-based protein.

17. **Kidney Beans:** Another nutritious option in the legume family.

18. **Pinto Beans:** High in protein and fiber.

19. **White Beans:** Mild in flavor and versatile in recipes.

20. **Quinoa:** A complete protein and an excellent grain alternative.

21. **Lean Beef (90% or Higher Lean):** Select lean cuts for lower fat content.

22. **Pork Tenderloin:** A lean cut of pork.

23. **Venison:** A game meat that is lean and rich in protein.

24. **Chicken or Turkey Sausages (Low Sodium):** Check labels for sodium content.

25. **Seitan:** A high-protein meat substitute made from gluten.

26. **Scallops:** Low in fat and a good source of protein.

27. **Crab:** A low-calorie and protein-rich seafood option.

28. **Mussels:** High in protein, vitamins, and minerals.

29. **Yogurt-Covered Nuts (Unsalted):** A protein-rich snack without added sodium.

30. **Whey Protein Isolate:** A low-fat, low-carb, and high-protein supplement.

Whole Grains

1. **Quinoa:** A versatile grain with a nutty flavor and a good source of protein.

2. **Brown Rice:** A whole grain with a chewy texture and nutty flavor.

3. **Oats:** High in fiber and perfect for breakfast as oatmeal or in baking.

4. **Buckwheat:** Despite its name, it's not wheat and is gluten-free.

5. **Barley:** Adds a chewy texture to soups and salads.

6. **Farro:** An ancient grain with a nutty flavor and chewy texture.

7. **Millet:** A small, round grain that's gluten-free and easy to digest.

8. **Amaranth:** High in protein and a good source of vitamins and minerals.

9. **Freekeh:** A roasted green wheat with a smoky flavor.

10. **Sorghum:** Gluten-free grain with a mild flavor, great for salads.

11. **Teff:** A tiny grain packed with nutrients, commonly used in Ethiopian cuisine.

12. **Wild Rice:** A nutrient-dense option with a hearty, chewy texture.

13. **Spelt:** An ancient grain with a nutty flavor and a good source of fiber.

14. **Bulgur:** A quick-cooking grain often used in Middle Eastern dishes.

15. **Whole Wheat Couscous:** A small pasta-like grain made from whole wheat.

16. **Brown Basmati Rice:** Fragrant long-grain rice with a nutty flavor.

17. **Whole Wheat Pasta:** A nutritious alternative to traditional pasta.

18. **Soba Noodles:** Buckwheat noodles that are popular in Japanese cuisine.

19. **Kamut:** An ancient grain with a rich, buttery flavor.

20. **Rye Berries:** Chewy, nutty grains that can be used in salads and side dishes.

21. **Whole Wheat Bulgur:** A whole grain form of cracked wheat, high in fiber.

22. **Sesame Seeds:** Tiny seeds rich in healthy fats and minerals.

23. **Sunflower Seeds:** Nutrient-packed seeds that add crunch to dishes.

24. **Chia Seeds:** High in omega-3 fatty acids and great for puddings and smoothies.

25. **Flaxseeds:** A good source of fiber and omega-3 fatty acids.

26. **Popcorn:** A whole grain snack when prepared without excessive salt.

27. **Bran Flakes:** High-fiber cereal that can be a nutritious breakfast option.

28. **Whole Wheat Bread:** Look for varieties with lower sodium content.

29. **Buckwheat Pancakes:** A tasty and nutritious breakfast option.

30. **Whole Grain Crackers:** Choose varieties with minimal added salt.

Dairy and Alternatives
Dairy

1. **Low-Fat or Fat-Free Milk:** An excellent source of calcium and vitamin D with lower sodium content.

2. **Greek Yogurt (Unflavored):** A protein-rich option with less sodium compared to some flavored varieties.

3. **Cottage Cheese (Low-Sodium):** Choose varieties labeled as low-sodium for reduced sodium content.

4. **Plain Yogurt:** Opt for plain, unsweetened yogurt to avoid added sodium found in flavored options.

5. **Mozzarella Cheese:** A lower-sodium cheese option that works well in various dishes.

Alternatives

6. **Almond Milk (Unsweetened):** A dairy-free, low-sodium milk alternative.

7. **Soy Milk (Unsweetened):** Another plant-based milk option with minimal sodium.

8. **Coconut Milk (Unsweetened):** Suitable for those looking for a dairy-free and low-sodium alternative.

9. **Oat Milk (Unsweetened):** A popular milk substitute with a naturally lower sodium content.

10. **Rice Milk (Unsweetened):** A low-sodium alternative for those with dairy allergies.

Non-Dairy Yogurt

11. **Coconut Yogurt (Unsweetened):** A dairy-free, low-sodium yogurt option.

12. **Almond Milk Yogurt (Unsweetened):** Rich in flavor and low in sodium.

13. **Soy Milk Yogurt (Unsweetened):** A plant-based yogurt with lower sodium content.

Cheese Alternatives

14. **Nutritional Yeast:** Adds a cheesy flavor to dishes with minimal sodium.

15. **Cashew Cheese:** A dairy-free option with lower sodium than some traditional cheeses.

16. **Vegan Parmesan:** A plant-based alternative with reduced sodium.

Other Alternatives

17. **Buttermilk (Low-Sodium):** Choose low-sodium varieties for a tangy flavor.

18. **Lactose-Free Milk:** A suitable option for those with lactose intolerance, often with lower sodium.

19. **Kefir (Low-Sodium):** A fermented dairy product with potential probiotic benefits.

Homemade Options:

20. **Homemade Yogurt:** Control the sodium content by making yogurt at home.

21. **Homemade Almond Milk:** Customize your almond milk with minimal sodium.

22. **Homemade Cashew Cheese:** Create a low-sodium cheese alternative at home.

Specialty Products:

23. **Low-Sodium Feta Cheese:** A reduced-sodium version of traditional feta.

24. **Low-Sodium Swiss Cheese:** A flavorful cheese with lower sodium content.

25. **Low-Sodium Blue Cheese:** A milder blue cheese option with reduced sodium.

International Options

26. **Paneer:** A type of Indian cheese with relatively low sodium.

27. **Labneh:** A Middle Eastern strained yogurt with potential lower sodium content.

28. **Queso Fresco:** A fresh Mexican cheese with a mild taste and moderate sodium.

Vegan Options

29. **Vegan Cream Cheese (Low-Sodium):** A dairy-free alternative with reduced sodium.

30. **Vegan Sour Cream (Low-Sodium):** A plant-based option for various recipes.

Herbs and Spices

1. Basil

2. Thyme

3. Oregano

4. Rosemary

5. Cilantro (Coriander)

6. Parsley

7. Sage

8. Mint

9. Dill

10. Chives

11. Tarragon

12. Bay Leaves

13. Cumin

14. Coriander

15. Paprika

16. Turmeric

17. Cinnamon

18. Nutmeg

19. Ginger

20. Garlic Powder

21. Onion Powder

22. Smoked Paprika

23. Cayenne Pepper

24. Mustard Powder

25. Chili Powder

26. Fennel Seeds

27. Cardamom

28. Allspice

29. Celery Seeds

30. Lemon Zest

Nuts and Seeds

Nuts

1. Almonds

2. Walnuts

3. Pecans

4. Hazelnuts

5. Pistachios

6. Cashews (in moderation, as they are higher in sodium than some other nuts)

7. Brazil nuts

8. Macadamia nuts

9. Pine nuts

10. Peanuts (unsalted)

Seeds

11. Chia seeds

12. Flaxseeds

13. Sunflower seeds (unsalted)

14. Pumpkin seeds (unsalted)

15. Sesame seeds

16. Hemp seeds

17. Poppy seeds

18. Watermelon seeds

19. Sunflower butter (unsalted)

20. Tahini (sesame seed paste)

Nut and Seed Mixes

21. Mixed nuts (unsalted)

22. Trail mix with unsalted nuts and seeds

23. Almond butter (unsalted)

24. Peanut butter (unsalted)

25. Cashew butter (unsalted)

26. Sunflower seed butter (unsalted)

Low Sodium Snacks with Nuts and Seeds

27. Rice cakes with almond butter

28. Nut and seed bars (check labels for low sodium options)

29. Homemade granola with unsalted nuts and seeds

30. Greek yogurt with a sprinkle of chia seeds and sliced almonds

How to overcome Challenges Adopting a Low Sodium Lifestyle

Dealing with Cravings

One of the most difficult aspects of adopting a low sodium diet is dealing with cravings for salty foods. To overcome these urges, you must be strategic and mindful:

1. Understanding the Root Cause

- Recognize that cravings are frequently the result of habit, emotional triggers, or conditioned responses to certain meals. Identifying the fundamental reason is the first step in properly managing cravings.

2. Gradual Reduction and Replacement

- Instead of going cold turkey, reduce sodium intake gradually to allow taste buds to acclimate. Replace salty snacks with healthy options like fresh fruits, unsalted almonds, or veggies with hummus.

3. Experimenting with Flavors

- Use herbs, spices, and other ingredients to improve the flavor of your meals. Experimenting with different flavors can satisfy the palate and reduce the craving for excessive salt.

4. Hydration

- Staying hydrated might aid in the reduction of cravings. When the body is thirsty, it will sometimes signal for salt. Drinking water throughout the day can help to reduce the desire for salty snacks.

5. Mindful Eating

- Staying hydrated might aid in the reduction of cravings. When the body is thirsty, it will sometimes signal for salt. Drinking water throughout the day can help to reduce the desire for salty snacks.

Navigating Social Situations

For individuals committed to a low salt lifestyle, social gatherings and dining out can present problems. Planning and effective communication are required to successfully navigate these situations:

1. Preparing in Advance

- Communicate food requirements to hosts or restaurant staff before attending social events. Bring a low sodium meal to share to ensure there are options that correspond with your dietary objectives.

2. Educating Friends and Family

- Take the time to educate your friends and family about the benefits of a low sodium diet for your health. They are more likely to be sympathetic and accommodating if they understand the reasons for your choices.

3. Choosing Wisely at Restaurants

- When dining out, examine restaurant menus ahead of time and select items that are likely to be lower in sodium. Request changes, such as requesting sauces on the side or choosing grilled over fried options.

4. Bringing Your Own Seasonings

- Bring a small jar of your favorite low sodium seasonings or sauces with you. This ensures that you may add taste to your meals even when dining out without relying on high-sodium condiments.

5. Focus on the Company

- Instead of focusing exclusively on the food, emphasize the social side of gatherings. Engaging in meaningful conversations and enjoying one's company can help to divert attention away from food constraints.

Staying Committed to a Low Sodium Lifestyle

Maintaining commitment to a low sodium lifestyle requires perseverance and the cultivation of healthy habits. Here are strategies to help stay on track:

1. Setting Realistic Goals

- Set attainable short-term and long-term goals. Gradual adjustments are more sustainable, and each modest win helps to the development of long-term habits.

2. Building a Support System

- Surround yourself with a supportive network of friends, family, or a community that shares similar health goals; having a support system gives encouragement and accountability.

3. Regular Check-Ins

- Evaluate your development on a regular basis. Reflecting on one's accomplishments and finding areas for development can assist to strengthen one's dedication and motivation.

4. Creating a Structured Meal Plan

- Plan meals ahead of time to ensure a balance of nutrients and flavors. A well-planned meal plan decreases the probability of relying on convenient, high-sodium choices.

5. Celebrating Milestones

- Celebrate all milestones, no matter how tiny they are. Recognize your accomplishments and reward yourself in non-food-related ways to reinforce the benefits of a low salt diet.

6. Learning from Setbacks

- Recognize that setbacks will occur and see them as opportunities to learn and adjust. Analyze the causes that contributed to the setback and put plans in place to deal with similar problems in the future.

CHAPTER 1

Breakfast Recipes

1. Avocado and Tomato Omelette

Ingredients

- 2 eggs

- 1/4 cup diced tomatoes

- 1/4 cup diced avocado

- Herbs such as chives or parsley can be use

- Salt-free seasoning

Preparation

- Whisk eggs and pour into a non-stick pan.
- Add tomatoes, avocados, and herbs.
- Cook until eggs are set. Season with salt-free seasoning.

Nutritional Information

- Calories: 250
- Protein: 14g
- Fat: 19g

- Carbohydrates: 8g

Serving Size: 1 omelette

Preparation Time: 10 minutes

2. Greek Yogurt Parfait

Ingredients

- 1 cup plain Greek yogurt

- 1/2 cup fresh berries

- 1 tablespoon chia seeds

- 1 tablespoon honey (optional)

Preparation

- In a glass, layer Greek yogurt, berries, chia seeds, and repeat.
- Drizzle with honey if desired.

Nutritional Information

- Calories: 220
- Protein: 20g
- Fat: 8g

- Carbohydrates: 18g

Serving Size: 1 parfait

Preparation Time: 5 minutes

3. Sweet Potato and Spinach Frittata

Ingredients

- 2 eggs

- 1/2 cup cooked sweet potatoes, diced

- 1 cup fresh spinach

- 1/4 cup diced onions

- Salt-free seasoning

Preparation

- Sauté onions and spinach until wilted.
- Whisk eggs and mix in sweet potatoes, spinach, and onions.
- It should be poured into a greased baking dish and bake until set.

Nutritional Information

- Calories: 280
- Protein: 16g
- Fat: 18g
- Carbohydrates: 15g

Serving Size: 1/4 frittata

Preparation Time: 20 minutes

4. Quinoa Breakfast Bowl

Ingredients

- 1/2 cup cooked quinoa
- 1/4 cup sliced almonds
- 1/2 cup fresh berries
- 1 tablespoon honey (optional)

Preparation

- Mix cooked quinoa with almonds and top with berries.
- Drizzle with honey if desired.

Nutritional Information

- Calories: 300
- Protein: 10g
- Fat: 12g
- Carbohydrates: 40g

Serving Size: 1 bowl

Preparation Time: 15 minutes

5. Spinach and Mushroom Breakfast Wrap

Ingredients

- 1 whole-grain tortilla

- 2 eggs, scrambled

- 1/2 cup fresh spinach

- 1/4 cup sliced mushrooms

- Salt-free seasoning

Preparation

- Sauté mushrooms until tender, then add spinach.
- Fill tortilla with scrambled eggs, spinach, and mushrooms.
- Season with salt-free seasoning.

Nutritional Information

- Calories: 280
- Protein: 15g
- Fat: 12g
- Carbohydrates: 30g

Serving Size: 1 wrap

Preparation Time: 10 minutes

6. Banana and Almond Butter Smoothie

Ingredients

- 1 banana
- 2 tablespoons almond butter
- 1 cup unsweetened almond milk
- Ice cubes

Preparation

- Blend banana, almond butter, almond milk, and ice until smooth.

Nutritional Information

- Calories: 300
- Protein: 7g
- Fat: 18g
- Carbohydrates: 30g

Serving Size: 1 smoothie

Preparation Time: 5 minutes

7. Oatmeal with Fresh Fruit

Ingredients

- 1/2 cup rolled oats
- 1 cup water or milk
- 1/2 cup sliced strawberries
- 1/4 cup blueberries
- Chopped nuts of 1 Table spoon (e.g., almonds or walnuts)

Preparation

- Cook oats with water or milk.
- Top with fresh fruit and chopped nuts.

Nutritional Information

- Calories: 250
- Protein: 8g
- Fat: 10g
- Carbohydrates: 35g

Serving Size: 1 bowl

Preparation Time: 10 minutes

8. Cottage Cheese and Pineapple Bowl

Ingredients

- 1/2 cup low-sodium cottage cheese
- 1/2 cup fresh pineapple chunks
- 1 tablespoon shredded coconut (unsweetened)

Preparation

- Mix cottage cheese with pineapple chunks.
- Sprinkle with shredded coconut.

Nutritional Information

- Calories: 180
- Protein: 15g
- Fat: 6g
- Carbohydrates: 20g

Serving Size: 1 bowl

Preparation Time: 5 minutes

9. Egg and Vegetable Muffins

Ingredients

- 4 eggs
- 1/2 cup diced bell peppers
- 1/4 cup diced tomatoes
- 1/4 cup chopped spinach
- Salt-free seasoning

Preparation

- Whisk eggs and mix in vegetables and seasoning.
- Pour into muffin tins and bake until set.

Nutritional Information

- Calories: 220
- Protein: 18g
- Fat: 14g
- Carbohydrates: 8g

Serving Size: 2 muffins

Preparation Time: 25 minutes

10. Smoked Salmon and Cream Cheese Bagel

Ingredients

- 1 whole-grain bagel, toasted
- 2 ounces smoked salmon
- 2 tablespoons low-fat cream cheese
- Fresh dill (optional)

Preparation

- The cream cheese should be spread on the toasted bagel.
- Top with smoked salmon and garnish with fresh dill if desired.

Nutritional Information

- Calories: 350
- Protein: 20g
- Fat: 12g
- Carbohydrates: 40g

Serving Size: 1 bagel

Preparation Time: 10 minutes

CHAPTER 2

Lunch Recipes

1. Grilled Lemon Herb Chicken Salad

Ingredients

- Boneless, skinless chicken breasts
- Mixed salad greens
- Cherry tomatoes
- Cucumber
- Red onion
- Lemon juice
- Olive oil
- Fresh herbs (such as parsley, thyme, or dill)

Preparation

- Season chicken with herbs, lemon juice, and a touch of olive oil.
- Grill until fully cooked.
- Toss grilled chicken with salad greens, cherry tomatoes, sliced cucumber, and red onion.

Nutritional Information

- Calories: 300
- Protein: 25
- Carbohydrates:10g
- Fat: 15g
- Sodium: 80mg

Serving Size: 1 serving

Preparation Time: 20 minutes

2. Quinoa and Vegetable Stuffed Peppers

Ingredients

- Bell peppers

- Quinoa

- Black beans (low-sodium or no-salt-added)

- Corn (fresh or frozen)

- Diced tomatoes (no salt added)

- Cumin, paprika, and garlic powder for seasoning

Preparation

- Cook quinoa according to package instructions.
- Mix quinoa with black beans, corn, diced tomatoes, and seasonings.
- Stuff bell peppers with the quinoa mixture and bake until peppers are tender.

Nutritional Information

- Calories: 250
- Protein: 8g
- Carbohydrates: 45g
- Fat: 4g
- Sodium: 50mg

Serving Size: 2 peppers (1 serving)

Preparation Time: 30 minutes

3. Salmon and Asparagus Foil Packets

Ingredients

- Salmon fillets

- Asparagus spears

- Lemon slices

- Fresh dill

- Olive oil

- Garlic (minced)

Preparation

- Place salmon fillets on foil, surround with asparagus.
- Drizzle with olive oil, add minced garlic, and top with lemon slices and fresh dill.
- Seal foil packets and bake until salmon is cooked through.

Nutritional Information

- Calories: 280
- Protein: 30g
- Carbohydrates: 5g

- Fat: 15g
- Sodium: 60mg

Serving Size: 1 packet

Preparation Time: 25 minutes

4. Turkey and Avocado Wrap

Ingredients

- Whole-grain tortilla
- Turkey breast slices (low-sodium)
- Avocado slices
- Spinach leaves
- Tomato slices
- Mustard for flavor

Preparation

- Spread mustard on the tortilla.
- Layer turkey slices, avocado, spinach, and tomato on the tortilla.
- Wrap and enjoy!

Nutritional Information

- Calories: 350
- Protein: 20g
- Carbohydrates: 30g
- Fat: 18g
- Sodium: 150mg

Serving Size: 1 wrap

Preparation Time: 10 minutes

5. Vegetarian Lentil Soup

Ingredients

- Lentils
- Carrots
- Celery
- Onion
- Garlic
- Vegetable broth (low-sodium)
- Cumin, coriander, and bay leaves for seasoning

Preparation

- Sauté onions, garlic, carrots, and celery in a pot.
- Add lentils, vegetable broth, and seasonings.
- Simmer until lentils and vegetables are tender.

Nutritional Information

- Calories: 220
- Protein: 15g
- Carbohydrates: 40g
- Fat: 1g
- Sodium: 80mg

Serving Size: 1.5 cups

Preparation Time: 40 minutes

6. Shrimp and Avocado Salad

Ingredients

- Shrimp (cooked and peeled)
- Avocado
- Cherry tomatoes
- Cilantro

- Lime juice

- Olive oil

- Salt-free seasoning

Preparation

- Combine shrimp, diced avocado, halved cherry tomatoes, and chopped cilantro.
- Drizzle with lime juice and olive oil. Season with salt-free seasoning.
- Toss gently and serve.

Nutritional Information

- Calories: 280
- Protein: 20g
- Carbohydrates: 10g
- Fat: 18g
- Sodium: 90mg

Serving Size: 1 cup

Preparation Time: 15 minutes

7. Vegetable Stir-Fry with Tofu

Ingredients

- Tofu
- Broccoli
- Bell peppers
- Snap peas
- Carrots
- Low-sodium soy sauce
- Ginger and garlic for flavor

Preparation

- The Tofu should be pressed and cubed, then stir-fry until golden.
- Add vegetables and stir-fry until tender-crisp.
- Low-sodium soy sauce, ginger, and garlic should be use for seasoning.

Nutritional Information

- Calories: 230
- Protein: 15g

- Carbohydrates: 20g

- Fat: 10g

- Sodium: 120mg

Serving Size: 1.5 cups

Preparation Time: 25 minutes

8. Chicken and Vegetable Brown Rice Bowl

Ingredients

- Chicken breast strips

- Broccoli

- Bell peppers

- Carrots

- Brown rice

- Low-sodium teriyaki sauce

- Sesame seeds for garnish

Preparation

- Cook chicken strips and set aside.
- Stir-fry vegetables until crisp-tender.

- Combine with cooked brown rice, add chicken, and drizzle with low-sodium teriyaki sauce. Garnish with sesame seeds.

Nutritional Information

- Calories: 300
- Protein: 25g
- Carbohydrates: 40g
- Fat: 5g
- Sodium: 140mg

Serving Size: 1.5 cups

Preparation Time: 30 minutes

9. Mushroom and Spinach Omelette

Ingredients

- Eggs
- Mushrooms
- Spinach
- Onion
- Low-fat cheese (optional)

- Herbs and spices for seasoning

Preparation

- Sauté mushrooms, spinach, and onions until cooked.
- Whisk eggs and pour over the vegetables in a pan.
- Cook until eggs are set, folding in half. Add optional cheese.

Nutritional Information (per serving)

- Calories: 220
- Protein: 18g
- Carbohydrates: 5g
- Fat: 15g
- Sodium: 180mg

Serving Size: 1 omelette

Preparation Time: 15 minutes

CHAPTER 3

Dinner Recipes

1. Grilled Lemon Garlic Chicken

Ingredients

- Chicken breasts

- Fresh lemon juice

- Olive oil

- Garlic (minced)

- Rosemary (fresh or dried)

- Black pepper

Preparation

1. Marinate chicken in a mixture of 2 tbsp lemon juice, 1 tbsp olive oil, 2 cloves minced garlic, 1 tsp rosemary, and 1/2 tsp black pepper for 30 minutes.

2. Grill until fully cooked.

Nutritional Information

- Calories: 250

- Sodium: 80 mg

- Protein: 30 g

- Fat: 12 g

- Carbohydrates: 4 g

Serving Size: 1 grilled chicken breast
Preparation Time: 40 minutes

2. Baked Cod with Herbs

Ingredients

- Cod fillets

- Fresh parsley (chopped)

- Dill (fresh or dried)

- Lemon zest

- Olive oil

- Black pepper

Preparation

1. Cod fillets should be placed on a baking sheet.

2. Mix 2 tbsp chopped parsley, 1 tsp dill, lemon zest, 1 tbsp olive oil, and 1/2 tsp black pepper. Spread over cod.

3. Bake until fish flakes easily.

Nutritional Information

- Calories: 180

- Sodium: 50 mg

- Protein: 22 g

- Fat: 8 g

- Carbohydrates: 2 g

Serving Size: 1 cod fillet

Preparation Time: 25 minutes

3. Vegetarian Quinoa Stuffed Peppers

Ingredients

- Bell peppers

- Quinoa

- Black beans (canned, rinsed)

- Corn

Preparation

1. Cook 1 cup quinoa. Mix with black beans and corn.

2. Stuff bell peppers with the quinoa mixture.

3. Bake until peppers are tender.

Nutritional Information

- Calories: 220

- Sodium: 20 mg

- Protein: 8 g

- Fat: 3 g

- Carbohydrates: 40 g

Serving Size: 1 stuffed pepper

Preparation Time: 45 minutes

4. Lemon Herb Grilled Shrimp Skewers

Ingredients

- Shrimp (peeled and deveined)

- Fresh lemon juice

- Olive oil

- Garlic (minced)

- Fresh parsley (chopped)

- Paprika

Preparation

1. Marinate shrimp in a mixture of 3 tbsp lemon juice, 2 tbsp olive oil, 2 cloves minced garlic, 2 tbsp chopped parsley, and 1 tsp paprika for 15 minutes.

2. The Shrimp should be thread onto skewers and grill until opaque.

Nutritional Information

- Calories: 150

- Sodium: 120 mg

- Protein: 20 g

- Fat: 7 g

- Carbohydrates: 2 g

Serving Size: 1 skewer

Preparation Time: 20 minutes

5. Mediterranean Chickpea Salad

Ingredients

- Chickpeas (canned, drained)

- Cherry tomatoes (halved)

- Cucumber (diced)

- Red onion (finely chopped)

- Kalamata olives (sliced)

- Feta cheese (crumbled)

- Olive oil

- Red wine vinegar

- Oregano

Preparation

1. Mix chickpeas, tomatoes, cucumber, red onion, olives, and feta in a bowl.

2. Drizzle with olive oil, red wine vinegar, and sprinkle with oregano. Toss to combine.

Nutritional Information

- Calories: 280

- Sodium: 400 mg

- Protein: 10 g

- Fat: 15 g

- Carbohydrates: 30 g

Serving Size: 1.5 cups

Preparation Time: 15 minutes

6. Lemon Dill Baked Chicken Thighs

Ingredients

- Chicken thighs (bone-in, skin-on)

- Fresh lemon juice

- Dill (fresh or dried)

- Garlic powder

- Olive oil

Preparation

1. Preheat the oven. Marinate chicken thighs in a mixture of lemon juice, dill, garlic powder, and olive oil.

2. Bake until the internal temperature reaches 165°F.

Nutritional Information

- Calories: 280

- Sodium: 80 mg

- Protein: 24 g

- Fat: 20 g

- Carbohydrates: 2 g

Serving Size: 2 chicken thighs

Preparation Time: 35 minutes

7. Baked Halibut with Tomato Salsa

Ingredients

- Halibut fillets

- Tomatoes (diced)

- Red onion (finely chopped)

- Cilantro (chopped)

- Lime juice

- Olive oil

- Salt and pepper to taste

Preparation

1. Preheat the oven. Place halibut fillets on a baking sheet.

2. In a bowl, mix tomatoes, red onion, cilantro, lime juice, olive oil, salt, and pepper.

3. Spoon salsa over halibut and bake until fish flakes easily.

Nutritional Information

- Calories: 220

- Sodium: 100 mg

- Protein: 30 g

- Fat: 10 g

- Carbohydrates: 5 g

Serving Size: 1 halibut fillet

Preparation Time: 30 minutes

8. Cauliflower and Chickpea Curry

Ingredients

- Cauliflower florets

- Chickpeas (canned, drained)

- Onion (chopped)

- Garlic (minced)

- Ginger (grated)

- Tomato sauce

- Coconut milk

- Curry powder

- Turmeric

- Cumin

- Coriander

- Salt and pepper to taste

Preparation:

1. Sauté onion, garlic, and ginger. Add cauliflower, chickpeas, tomato sauce, coconut milk, and spices.

2. Simmer until cauliflower is tender.

Nutritional Information

- Calories: 280

- Sodium: 300 mg

- Protein: 10 g

- Fat: 15 g

- Carbohydrates: 30 g

Serving Size: 1.5 cups

Preparation Time: 40 minutes

9. Turkey and Vegetable Skillet

Ingredients

- Ground turkey

- Bell peppers (sliced)

- Zucchini (sliced)

- Onion (chopped)

- Garlic (minced)

- Tomato sauce

- Italian seasoning

- Olive oil

- Salt and pepper to taste

Preparation

1. In a skillet, cook ground turkey. Add bell peppers, zucchini, onion, and garlic.

2. Stir in tomato sauce, Italian seasoning, salt, and pepper. Simmer until vegetables are tender.

Nutritional Information

- Calories: 250

- Sodium: 300 mg

- Protein: 20 g

- Fat: 12 g

- Carbohydrates: 15 g

Serving Size: 1 cup

Preparation Time: 30 minutes

10. Spinach and Feta Stuffed Chicken Breast

Ingredients

- Chicken breasts

- Spinach (fresh or frozen)

- Feta cheese (crumbled)

- Garlic (minced)

- Olive oil

- Lemon juice

- Salt and pepper to taste

Preparation

1. Preheat the oven. Sauté spinach and garlic in olive oil until wilted. Mix with feta cheese.

2. Cut a pocket in each chicken breast, stuff with spinach mixture, and drizzle with lemon juice.

3. Bake until chicken is cooked through.

Nutritional Information

- Calories: 280

- Sodium: 250 mg

- Protein: 30 g

- Fat: 12 g

- Carbohydrates: 8 g

Serving Size: 1 stuffed chicken breast

Preparation Time: 45 minutes

CHAPTER 4

7 days meal plan

Day 1

Breakfast- **Avocado and Tomato Omelette**

Lunch- **Grilled Lemon Herb Chicken Salad**

Dinner- **Grilled Lemon Garlic Chicken**

Day 2

Breakfast- **Greek Yogurt Parfait**

Lunch- **Quinoa and Vegetable Stuffed Peppers**

Dinner- **Baked Cod with Herbs**

Day 3

Breakfast- **Sweet Potato and Spinach Frittata**

Lunch- **Salmon and Asparagus Foil Packets**

Dinner- **Vegetarian Quinoa Stuffed Peppers**

Day 4

Breakfast- **Quinoa Breakfast Bowl**

Lunch- **Mushroom and Spinach Omelette**

Dinner- **Herb Grilled Shrimp Skewers**

Day 5

Breakfast- **Spinach and Mushroom Breakfast Wrap**

Lunch- **Turkey and Avocado Wrap**

Dinner- **Mediterranean Chickpea Salad**

Day 6

Breakfast- **Banana and Almond Butter Smoothie**

Lunch- **Vegetarian Lentil Soup**

Dinner- **Lemon Dill Baked Chicken Thighs**

Day 7

Breakfast- **Oatmeal with Fresh Fruit**

Lunch- **Shrimp and Avocado Salad**

Dinner- **Baked Halibut with Tomato Salsa**

CHAPTER 5

Conclusion

This is a complete guide to low-sodium living, it is clear that adopting a low-sodium lifestyle is a powerful and proactive step toward reaching and sustaining good health. Throughout these pages, we've looked at the complex meaning of low sodium diet and its profound impact on a variety of areas of health, from cardiovascular health to kidney function and beyond.

The quest began by delving into the science of sodium, providing light on its position in the body's complicated systems and the potential effects of excessive consumption. Following that, we dug into the far-reaching health hazards associated with high salt intake, emphasizing the critical importance of adopting a low-sodium diet as a cornerstone of preventative health care.

The heart of this guide took the form of practical and delectable low-sodium dishes that were precisely developed to excite the taste buds while keeping sodium content under control. Each recipe, from grilled lemon garlic chicken to Mediterranean chickpea salad, provided not just a gourmet joy but also a wholesome option geared at feeding the body from inside.

Readers are empowered to make informed decisions that extend beyond the constraints of a single meal after learning about the importance of low sodium living and receiving a compilation of scrumptious recipes. These choices have a significant impact on the avoidance of chronic diseases, the promotion of cardiovascular health, and the growth of overall well-being.

As we conclude this journey, let it serve as a beginning point rather than a finish. The core of low-sodium living is a lifestyle transformation, not just a food change—an ongoing commitment to prioritizing health and embracing the vigor that comes with it. Whether you're doing it for yourself, a loved one, or the entire community, the impacts of thoughtful and health-conscious choices are limitless.

May this guide serve as a guidepost on your path to a life of balance, flavor, and wellness. Accept the art of savoring each food, embrace the journey toward greater health, and relish the satisfaction that comes from knowing that every decision you make adds to a healthier and happy you.